OSTOMY BAG MAINTENANCE DIET

Complete Guide Unlocking The Secrets Of
Nutrition To Rapid Healing After Surgery
Success, Nourishing Meal Plans, Recipes, Tips
For Optimal Health Wellness

DR. ALLAN FREDA

Contents

INTRODUCTION

We're glad you found our guide to the Ostomy Bag Maintenance Diet. People who have had ostomy surgery or are getting ready for it should find this cookbook helpful.

It is full of useful information and recipes. Living with an ostomy bag can be hard in some ways, especially when it comes to food and nutrition.

However, it is possible to live a healthy and satisfying life with the right information and help.

This guide will go over the main ideas of the ostomy bag care diet, such as why food choices are important, what problems people often face, and how to deal with them in the best way possible.

This resource is meant to give you the tools you need to thrive, whether you are new to living with an ostomy or want to improve your food after surgery.

This guide is a collection of expert advice, real-life experience, and new recipes that are perfect for people who have ostomy bags. The result of working together with nutritionists, health care workers, and people who have had ostomy surgery themselves.

Our goal is to give you a complete resource that goes beyond simple dietary advice to meet the unique needs and problems that ostomates face. This cookbook takes a complete look at the ostomy bag maintenance diet, from explaining the importance of various nutrients to providing tasty and healthy food ideas. You will find useful information on these pages, whether you are looking for easy meal ideas, help with specific dietary issues, or health tips for the long term.

How to Understand the Ostomy Bag Maintenance Diet:

To stay healthy and happy while living with an ostomy bag, you need to be very careful about what you eat. During ostomy surgery, a stoma is made, which is an opening in the belly through which waste leaves the body and goes into a pouch or bag that is worn on the outside. This change in the digestive system can affect how food is digested, absorbed, and poop habits, which means that diet and lifestyle need to be changed.

The ostomy bag maintenance diet is meant to improve general health, keep the digestive system healthy, and stop problems like blockages or leaks. It means learning about the functions of different nutrients, figuring out which foods can make you feel bad or give you stomach problems, and making plans to keep your diet healthy and balanced.

A full guide to the best diet for people who have just had surgery or been diagnosed with a new illness. It includes healing recipes, meal plans, and expert advice for long-term health:

After ostomy surgery, it's important to keep track of your food and nutrition for healing, recovery, and long-term health. People who just found out they have an ostomy bag may feel overwhelmed by the thought of adjusting to life with one, which may include making changes to their food.

This complete guide is meant to help people get on the right track for a healthy diet after surgery and long-term fitness by giving them step-by-step instructions, healing recipes, customisable meal plans, and expert advice. People can speed up the healing process, avoid complications, and enjoy a varied and satisfying diet that feeds both body and soul by adding nutrient-rich foods, limiting possible triggers, and practicing mindful eating. This guide has recipes for everything from healthy salads and main dishes to comforting soups and smoothies. The recipes are not only tasty but they are also meant to help your digestive health and general health. This guide is meant to give you the information and tools you need to thrive after ostomy surgery, whether you are looking for practical tips on how to deal with common problems like controlling gas or smells or ideas for tasty and healthy meals. People who have an ostomy and want to live a healthier and happier life will find this guide very helpful. It focuses on holistic wellness and personalized care.

Disclaimer

The information in this book is for informational purposes only and should not replace professional medical advice, diagnosis, or treatment. Always consult your physician or a qualified health provider regarding any medical concerns. Do not disregard professional medical advice or delay seeking it based on information in this book.

The author does not endorse or have affiliations with any mentioned entities. References are for informational purposes only.

Consult your healthcare provider before making dietary or lifestyle changes, especially during recovery from surgery, as individual needs vary.

Results may vary, and the information provided is not guaranteed to produce specific outcomes.

By reading this book, you acknowledge and agree to consult your healthcare provider before implementing any information herein.

For further guidance, consult your healthcare provider or reputable medical websites for reliable information on surgery recovery diets.

CHAPTER 1

GETTING STARTED

Important Tools and Equipment

When you start an ostomy bag maintenance diet, it's very important to have the right tools and equipment to make sure you stay comfortable, keep yourself clean, and handle your condition well. These tools not only make the process easier, but they also improve your health and give you more confidence in your ability to take care of your ostomy.

Ostomy pouches, which come in different styles like one-piece or two-piece sets, are very important tools. One-piece systems have a pouch and adhesive that are combined, while two-piece systems have different pouches and adhesive barriers. This means that you can change the pouch without taking the whole appliance off. Stoma measure guides also help make sure that the pouching system is the right size and fits your stoma properly, which stops leaks and pain. If you want to cut bags to fit your stoma perfectly without hurting yourself, you need ostomy scissors with rounded tips. Using skin barrier wipes or sprays around the stoma protects it from itching and helps keep the skin healthy. Stoma powder and paste help keep the skin from getting irritated and keep the ostomy device securely in place. Lastly, adhesive removers help gently loosen and remove the adhesive without hurting the skin. This makes it easier to change pouches with little pain.

Putting food in your pantry

To stick to a healthy ostomy bag care diet, you need to make sure your pantry is always stocked. Your pantry should have a variety of healthy foods that are good for your digestive system, keep you from having problems with your ostomy, and improve your general health.

Fiber-rich foods, like whole grains, fruits, and veggies, are important for keeping bowel movements regular and avoiding constipation, which is a common problem for people with ostomies. But it's important to add fiber slowly and keep an eye on how it affects your digestive system since too much fiber can cause clogs or more gas production. Lean proteins, like those found in chicken, fish, tofu, and legumes, help fix damaged tissues and keep muscles strong without making ostomy output worse.

Adding probiotic-rich foods like yogurt, kefir, and fermented greens to your diet can help keep the balance of bacteria in your gut healthy and lower your risk of pouch smell and infection.

Also, staying hydrated is important to avoid becoming dehydrated and to keep your stomach working well, so make sure you stock up on water, herbal teas, and drinks that are high in electrolytes. Lastly, keep low-residue snacks like rice cakes, crackers, and smooth nut butter on hand for times when you need something light and easy to digest.

Learning the Basics of Ostomies

To fully understand an ostomy bag maintenance diet, it is important to first have a solid grasp of the basic principles of ostomy care and management. An ostomy is a surgically made opening in the abdomen that lets waste leave the body when the regular way of doing so is blocked, like in people with colorectal cancer, inflammatory bowel disease, or trauma.

The three main types of ostomies are colostomy, ileostomy, and urostomy. Each one is used for a different reason depending on where the stoma is located and the underlying medical condition.

A colostomy moves part of the colon to the surface of the abdomen. This usually makes the stool thicker and more solid. Because the colon isn't working, the ileostomy moves the small intestine to the abdominal wall. This makes the stool more liquid because the colon isn't absorbing food. If you have a urostomy, on the other hand, urine goes from the bladder to a stoma on the belly.

This means you need a different pouching system that is made just for collecting urine. Knowing the type of ostomy you have and what it does is important for managing it properly and following dietary rules that are made just for you. To stay comfortable and avoid problems, it's also important to know how to take care of your stoma, including good cleanliness, skin protection, and how to fix common problems like leakage or irritation.

By learning the basics of ostomy care, you can face the challenges of living with an ostomy with confidence and improve your quality of life as a whole.

How to Make Foods That Are Good for People with Ostomies

Ostomy surgery is a life-changing procedure that includes making a hole in the abdomen so that waste can drain into a pouch, which is called an ostomy bag. People who have had ostomy surgery may need to change what they eat to make sure their digestive system is comfortable and their health is better overall. This complete guide will talk about the rules of ostomy-friendly food, what ostomy patients should eat, and how to cook in a way that makes digestion easier.

How to Cook for People with Ostomies

When cooking for someone with an ostomy, there are a few things you should keep in mind to make sure their digestive health and general health are at their best. To begin, it's important to focus on eating things that are easy for the digestive system to break down. This means making sure meals have a lot of cooked fruits and veggies, lean proteins, and whole grains.

Also, watching the size of your portions can help keep you from getting stomachaches and other problems.

Instead of big, heavy meals several times a day, eating smaller meals more often can help digestion and keep the ostomy bag from getting too full or heavy.

Ostomy patients also need to make sure they stay properly hydrated. Dehydration can be avoided by drinking a lot of water throughout the day.

This is especially important for people with an ostomy, who may lose more fluids than others.

In addition, it's important to know which foods can give you gas, bloating, or other stomach problems. Some of these are carbonated drinks, foods high in fiber like broccoli and beans, and meals that are very spicy or have a lot of seasoning. Avoiding these foods or eating them in small amounts can help keep stomach problems from happening.

When cooking for someone with an ostomy, it's important to choose foods that are gentle and easy to digest, watch your amount size, stay hydrated, and be aware of foods that may cause digestive discomfort.

People who have an ostomy need to make sure they eat right to help their bodies heal, avoid problems, and improve their general health and well-being. Some people who have had ostomy surgery may have changes in how they digest and absorb nutrients. Because of this, it is important to focus on eating foods that are high in nutrients and provide necessary vitamins and minerals.

Making sure that ostomy people get enough protein is one of the most important nutritional issues they need to think about. Protein is needed to mend tissues and heal wounds, which makes it even more important for people who have recently had surgery. Chicken, fish, eggs, tofu, and beans are all lean sources of protein that can be added to meals to help with healing and recovery.

It's also important for people with ostomies to eat enough fiber to keep their gut systems healthy. Some people may need to avoid high-fiber foods right after surgery to keep their intestines from getting clogged, but slowly adding them back into your diet can help prevent constipation and encourage normal bowel movements. Dietary fiber can be found in whole grains, fruits, veggies, nuts, and seeds.

Also, people with ostomies may need to watch how much vitamin B12, calcium, and iron they take in. People may not get enough of these nutrients depending on the type of ostomy surgery they had and any other health problems they may already have. Foods that are high in these vitamins and minerals, like dairy products, leafy veggies, lean meats, and fortified cereals, can help keep you from falling short and improve your health as a whole.

Overall, ostomy patients should focus on eating protein-rich foods to help their bodies heal, slowly reintroducing fibre to support digestive health, and making sure they get enough important vitamins and minerals to avoid deficiencies and improve their overall health.

Techniques for cooking that are good for digestion

Along with choosing the right foods, there are ways to cook that can help people with an ostomy feel better when they are digesting. One of the most important things to think about is how to cook foods so that they are easy to digest. For example, instead of frying or grilling, foods may need to be steamed, boiled, or baked. These cooking methods can help break down tough fibers and make foods more tender and easier to swallow.

Using herbs and spices in cooking can also make food taste better without using heavy sauces or seasonings which can make your stomach hurt. Herbs like parsley, basil, and mint can make food taste fresh, and spices like turmeric and ginger can help your digestive system feel better and reduce swelling.

If you are cooking for someone with an ostomy, you should also pay attention to the food's temperature. Extremely hot or cold foods and drinks can hurt your stomach and make you feel uncomfortable. Try to give food at a moderate temperature to avoid any problems.

People with an ostomy must also follow proper food hygiene and safety steps to avoid getting sick from food and having digestive problems. This means washing fruits and veggies well, cooking meats to the right temperature, and storing leftovers in the right way to keep them from getting dirty.

To improve the general health of people with an ostomy, cooking techniques for digestive comfort include using gentle cooking methods, adding herbs and spices for flavor, serving foods at moderate temperatures, and making sure they are clean and safe when handling food.

CHAPTER 3
IDEAS FOR BREAKFAST

Many people believe that breakfast is the most important meal of the day. This is especially true for people who have had ostomy surgery. A healthy diet is important for people who are getting used to living with an ostomy bag and want to heal as quickly as possible. In this in-depth guide to ostomy bag care diet, we'll talk about how to make a post-surgery diet plan that helps you heal, makes sure you get enough nutrition and supports your long-term health. Breakfast is an important part of this diet plan because it sets the tone for the day and gives the body the nutrients it needs to run.

Here, we'll talk about different breakfast ideas that are good for people with an ostomy, such as quick and easy options, high-protein options, and creative recipes that will make the morning meal more fun and interesting.

Breakfasts that are quick and easy:

After ostomy surgery, people may have changes in their energy levels and need easy food options that don't take much time to make. Breakfasts that are quick and easy are great for busy mornings or when you're feeling tired because they give you the nutrition you need without a lot of work.

Overnight oats are one choice. They are a healthy and flexible dish that can be made ahead of time and changed to fit each person's tastes. Rolling oats can be mixed with milk or yogurt and toppings like nuts, seeds, veggies, and other foods to make a healthy breakfast that is easy on the stomach and gives plenty of energy all morning. Also, smoothies are an easy way to get a lot of different minerals in one meal. People can make a healthy, refreshing breakfast that is easy to stomach on the go by mixing fruits, vegetables, protein sources like Greek yogurt or protein powder, and liquids like almond milk or coconut water.

A simple egg scramble with veggies is a quick and easy way to get protein, vitamins, and minerals for those who like savory foods. People can have a healthy breakfast in minutes by sautéing veggies like spinach, bell peppers, and tomatoes and then adding beaten eggs. These quick and easy breakfast ideas are great for people with an ostomy because they are easy to make and provide important nutrients without sacrificing taste or ease.

Breakfast Foods High in Protein:

Protein is an important part of the diet for people who have had surgery on an ostomy because it helps repair tissues and keep muscles strong. By offering high-protein breakfast choices, you can make sure that people get the protein they need while also helping them heal and recover.

Not only is Greek yogurt a great source of protein but it can also be eaten on its own or added to different breakfast meals. By mixing Greek yogurt with nuts, fruits, and honey, you can make a healthy, filling breakfast that is also easy on the stomach. Cottage cheese is another breakfast food that is high in protein. It can be eaten plain or mixed with fruits or veggies to make it taste better and give you more nutrients. Eggs are also a flexible source of protein because they can be cooked in many ways, such as baked, boiled, or poached. When you eat eggs with whole grain toast or veggies for breakfast, you get a healthy, filling meal that helps your muscles recover. Tofu or tempeh can be used instead of animal nutrients for people who would rather eat plant-based foods. People with an ostomy can make sure they get enough protein for healing and general health by adding these high-protein breakfast options to their meal plans.

Unique Breakfast Ideas:

It's important to eat a variety of foods to keep your diet healthy and fun. This is especially true for people with special dietary needs, like those who have an ostomy. There are lots of creative ways to use healthy foods in breakfast recipes that keep meals interesting and tasty. A breakfast quinoa bowl is a creative way to start the day. It has cooked quinoa, veggies, nuts, seeds, and a drizzle of honey or maple syrup on top. Because it is high in protein, fiber, and important vitamins and minerals, this breakfast is a great choice for people who have an ostomy. Avocado toast is another creative way to start the day. It is made with whole grain bread, mashed avocado, and toppings like smoked salmon, tomatoes, or a fried egg. Whole-grain bread gives you fiber and energy that lasts, and avocado has good fats, vitamins, and minerals. If you like sweets, banana pancakes made with mashed bananas, eggs, and oat flour are a tasty and healthy alternative to regular pancakes. For people who are still getting used to living with an ostomy, these creative breakfast ideas are a great way to get the nutrients they need while also making the meal more interesting and varied.

breakfast is an important part of the ostomy bag care diet because it gives you the nutrients you need to heal, have energy, and be healthy in general. People with an ostomy can enjoy a varied and healthy breakfast that fits their dietary needs and tastes by planning their meals around quick and easy breakfasts, high-protein options, and creative recipes. With the right food choices and planning their meals, people with an ostomy can go through life with confidence and be healthy for a long time.

CHAPTER 4
DINNER AND LUNCH RECIPE

Ostomy bag maintenance food is very important for people who have had ostomy surgery to keep them healthy and improve their quality of life. This complete guide is meant to help people who are getting used to living with an ostomy bag figure out how to make a diet that helps them heal, improves their nutrition, and keeps them comfortable. This part goes over lunch and dinner meals that are made to fit the dietary needs of people who have ostomies.

Making Salads That Are Ostomy-Friendly:

People with ostomies can easily change salads to meet their food needs because they are very flexible. When making salads that are good for people with ostomies, it's important to choose vegetables that are easy on the digestive system and won't hurt or irritate it. Leafy greens, like spinach or kale, are good for you because they are low in calories and high in minerals. Adding low-residue veggies like bell peppers, shredded carrots, and cucumber will add texture and flavor without making blockages more likely. Adding lean protein sources like grilled chicken, tofu, or hard-boiled eggs to the salad will make it healthier. Don't use high-fiber foods like nuts, seeds, or raw cruciferous veggies because they might be hard to digest and could make problems with your ostomy worse. Use a light vinegar or olive oil-based dressing to add flavor to the salad without making it too heavy for your stomach. Try putting together different kinds of vegetables in different ways to make tasty, healthy salads that people with ostomies can eat.

Sandwiches and wraps that fill you up:
People who have ostomies can easily change the ingredients in sandwiches and wraps to make them fit their food needs. For ostomy-friendly meals like sandwiches and wraps, it's important to use soft bread or wraps that are easy to swallow. If

you want to avoid getting clogged up and feeling bad, choose whole-grain or white bread that is low in fiber.

Lean protein sources, like sliced turkey, chicken, or fish, should be used as fillings because they provide important nutrients without too much fat or fiber. Add lettuce, tomatoes, avocado, and other moisturizing foods to your food to make it taste and feel better without making your stomach upset.

Do not use items that are high in fiber or hard to digest, like raw vegetables, seeds, or crunchy nuts. Spread a thin layer of hummus or low-fat mayonnaise on the bread or wrap to make it more flavorful and moister. You can make tasty sandwiches and wraps that are easy on the stomach and good for people with ostomies by trying out different fillings and toppings.

Healthy Soups and Stews:

Soups and stews are comfortable and healthy meals that can be changed to fit the needs of people who have ostomies. When making soups and stews that are good for people with ostomies, it's important to use ingredients that are soft, easy to swallow, and not likely to irritate or hurt the person. Broth-based soups are better than cream-based soups because they are lighter and less likely to make problems with your ostomy worse.

Chicken, turkey, fish, and other lean protein sources should be on the menu, along with a range of vegetables that have been cooked until soft. Don't use broccoli, cauliflower, cabbage, or other high-fiber veggies because they might be hard to digest and cause digestive problems.

Thinking about adding cooked grains like rice or quinoa to the soup could make it healthier and give you energy at the same time. To make the soup or stew taste better without making you more likely to get sick, add herbs, spices, and low-sodium stock. Try putting different items together in new ways to make healthy soups and stews that people with ostomies can eat.

Lunch and dinner dishes with lots of flavor:

The main part of any meal is the entree, which can be changed to fit the needs of people with ostomies without affecting the taste or pleasure.

When making main dishes for ostomy-friendly meals, it's important to use lean protein sources, complex carbs, and foods that are easy on the digestive system. Choose meats that are grilled or baked, like chicken, fish, or tofu.

These foods provide important nutrients without too much fat or fiber. To give the dish more texture and body, serve the chicken with cooked grains like couscous, brown rice, or quinoa. Include a range of cooked veggies that are soft and easy to digest, like bell peppers, mushrooms, and zucchini. Don't use ingredients that are high in fiber or hard to digest, like cruciferous veggies, beans, or lentils. You could add herbs, spices, and fruits to the dish to make it taste better without making your stomach upset. Play around with different cooking methods and flavor combinations to come up with tasty main dishes that people with ostomies can eat.

For long-term health, it is important to make sure that people with ostomies have a diet that helps them heal, promotes nutrition, and keeps them comfortable. People can enjoy tasty and healthy meals without affecting their gut health by planning their meals around ostomy-friendly salads, filling sandwiches and wraps, healthy soups and stews, and flavorful main dishes. People who live with ostomies can make a varied and satisfying meal that meets their specific dietary needs if they pay close attention to the ingredients they use and how they cook them.

CHAPTER 5

SNACKS AND STARTERS

Snacks and appetizers are important parts of the ostomy bag maintenance diet because they help you keep up a healthy diet and meet the unique needs and challenges that may come up after surgery. These little bites are not only good for you, but they are also convenient, satisfying, and even good for socializing.

There are savory appetizers that are good for social events, portable snacks that can be eaten on the go, and guilt-free desserts that are all important for making sure that people with an ostomy stay healthy and happy. We talk about the importance of snacks and appetizers in the diet after surgery in this in-depth guide. It also includes healing recipes, meal plans, and expert tips for long-term health.

Snacks that you can take with you

People who have had ostomy surgery often have to get used to a new schedule, which may include making changes to the foods they eat.

Portable snacks become necessary friends because they keep you fed on busy days, while traveling, or just when you're not at home. Not only are these snacks easy to get, but they were also carefully picked to help your digestive health and keep you from having any problems or discomfort because of your ostomy bag.

Fruits, nuts, yogurt, and granola bars are all great choices because they are easy to swallow. Getting the right amount of carbs, proteins, and fats in your diet will keep your energy up and your health in general all day. Additionally, people can make snacks, like energy balls or trail mix, that suit their personal tastes and nutritional needs. People can stay healthy and independent while on the go by putting flexibility, digestibility, and nutritional value first.

Social events and meetings often center around food, which can be both helpful and difficult for people who have an ostomy.

To solve this problem, tasty appetizers are perfect because they let people eat with others without having to worry about their health or comfort. When choosing appetizers, people look for foods that are easy on the stomach but have a lot of flavor and texture.

Crudités of vegetables with hummus, grilled prawn skewers, or stuffed mushrooms are all great choices that can be made to fit a wide range of dietary needs and restrictions. Adding herbs and spices not only makes the food taste better, but they may also be good for you in some ways, like reducing inflammation or helping the digestive system.

By providing a variety of savory appetizers, hosts can make sure that all of their guests feel welcome and enjoy the event, even those who need to follow special dietary needs because of ostomy surgery.

Dessert Bites You Can Eat Without Feeling Bad

In many cooking customs, desserts have a special place because they represent celebration and overindulgence. But for people with an ostomy, it can be hard to choose a treat because they are worried about the ingredients that might make them feel bad or cause digestive problems.

These worries can be eased with guilt-free dessert bites, which offer tasty options that put digestive health first.

These desserts are made with healthy ingredients like nuts, fruits, and whole grains, and they don't have a lot of extra sugars or artificial ingredients. Fruit on sticks dipped in yogurt, dark chocolate-covered nuts or oatmeal cookies sweetened with natural ingredients are all examples.

People can enjoy dessert without feeling guilty or having digestive problems if they choose nutrient-dense foods and watch their portions. Additionally, trying new recipes and flavor combinations will make cooking more interesting and fun, which will help you stick to a healthy diet after surgery.

CHAPTER 6
MENUS FOR SPECIAL OCCASIONS

When dealing with an ostomy bag, eating a healthy diet is very important for your health and well-being as a whole. On holidays and other special days, there can be some unique problems, but there are also chances to enjoy tasty meals while meeting food needs. People with ostomies can still enjoy tasty foods without putting their health at risk at a family meeting, a holiday party, or a special event. This complete guide will talk about many different ways to make special occasion dinners that are perfect for people with ostomies. It includes holiday and event-themed meals, party-planning tips, and ideas for tasty treats to enjoy on these special days.

Holiday and event celebration meals:

People with ostomies need to carefully plan their meals, especially during holidays and events where food is a big deal. Even though it might seem hard at first, there are a lot of tasty and healthy choices that can work for everyone, no matter their likes or dietary needs. Planning holiday and event meals for people with ostomies should focus on including foods that are easy on the digestive system, don't cause pain or problems, and are gentle on the digestive system.

When planning festive meals, it's important to think about how to add a range of tastes and textures to make the experience better. Choose dishes that are high in nutrients, like fruits, veggies, lean proteins, and whole grains. Stay away from foods that may make your stomach hurt or give you digestive problems. Fiber-rich foods in moderation can also help control bowel movements and improve gut health. However, it's important to choose soluble fiber sources to keep the stoma from getting clogged.

When planning a celebration meal, lean meats like chicken, fish, tofu, and beans are great options. People who have ostomies can eat these proteins because they are easy to digest and less likely to make you gassy or bloated. It's also important to include a lot of veggies in holiday meals.

However, fibrous vegetables like broccoli, cabbage, and cauliflower should be avoided because they can make you feel uncomfortable and give you gas. Choose cooked or steamed veggies instead, like spinach, green beans, and carrots. They are better for your digestive system.

Throwing parties for people with ostomies:

Catering to people with special food needs can make it hard to host parties and other events, but with some planning and thought, it is possible to make sure that guests with ostomies feel welcome and included. Communication is very important when planning parties for people with ostomies.

Ask your guests ahead of time about any food restrictions or preferences they may have.

This will help you plan a meal that meets everyone's needs.

When planning the food for an ostomy-friendly party, make sure there are lots of different choices so that everyone can find something they like.

On your menu, make sure there are lots of fresh fruits and veggies, lean proteins, and whole grains. You might also want to make dishes that are easy to change to fit the needs of people with different dietary restrictions. Making sure there are a variety of appetizers, main courses, and desserts means that guests with ostomies can enjoy the party without thinking about being uncomfortable or having digestive problems.

When planning an ostomy-friendly party, it's important to think about more than just the menu. The way the food is served is also very important. Putting allergen information and ingredients on the labels of dishes can help guests make better food choices and lower the chance that they will eat something that makes them feel bad by mistake. Offering a range of serving plates and utensils can also help keep food from getting contaminated, protecting guests with special dietary needs.

Some people with ostomies can still enjoy these tasty treats with a few changes. No celebration is complete without festive treats and desserts. When choosing holiday treats, it's important to choose ones that are low in fat, sugar, and fiber to avoid stomach problems and pain. People who have ostomies can also enjoy special occasions without worrying about digestive problems by picking treats that are easy to digest and gentle on the digestive system.

When you make holiday treats for people with ostomies, you might want to use ingredients that are easy on the digestive system, like whole grains, ripe fruits, and low-fat dairy products.

High-fat foods, fake sweeteners, and too much fiber are some of the things that should be avoided if you want to avoid gas, bloating, or diarrhea. Instead, focus on using natural sweeteners like maple syrup or honey and flavors like cinnamon, vanilla, and lemon to make your treats taste better without adding extra calories or chemicals.

Fruit sticks with yogurt dip, homemade sorbets and fruit popsicles, and baked goods made with whole grains and natural sweeteners are all tasty holiday treats that are also safe for people with ostomies. Not only are these treats tasty, but they are also good for you because they contain vitamins, minerals, and antioxidants that are good for your general health and well-being. Adding holiday flavors and decorations can also make your treats feel more like the season, making them great for parties and other special events.

Finally, holidays and events are great times to enjoy tasty foods and treats while meeting dietary goals. People with ostomies can enjoy special occasions without putting their health or well-being at risk by making sure that celebratory meals are made with gentle and healthy ingredients, throwing parties that are accessible to people with ostomies, and making holiday treats that are easy to digest. Planning and giving things some thought can help you make great dining experiences that meet everyone's wants and needs. This way, everyone can enjoy the party and celebrate in style.

CHAPTER 7
DRINKS AND SMOOTHIES

Smoothies and drinks are an important part of an ostomy patient's diet because they help them stay hydrated and provide nutrition and comfort.

After ostomy surgery, it's important to stay properly hydrated for a speedy recovery and general health. Electrolyte changes, kidney problems, and less energy are some of the problems that can happen when you're dehydrated. Besides that, some drinks and shakes can give you important vitamins and nutrients that help your body heal and stay healthy over time.

This complete guide to the best post-surgery diet for people who have just been labeled with an ostomy talks about how important it is to stay hydrated and gives smoothie recipes and other drink ideas that are specifically made for people with ostomies.

Ostomy patients must stay properly hydrated to stay healthy and avoid problems. However, people with ostomies may have trouble staying properly hydrated because they lose more fluids through the stoma. Here are some important tips for ostomy people on how to stay hydrated:

1. Watch How Much You Drink: Make sure you're drinking enough water by keeping track of how much you drink throughout the day. Aim to drink eight 8-ounce glasses of water every day, but this can change depending on your exercise level, the weather, and your health.

2. Pick drinks that have a lot of vitamins in them. Electrolytes are minerals like magnesium, potassium, and sodium that help the body keep the right mix of fluids. Electrolyte-rich drinks like coconut water, sports drinks, and electrolyte-enhanced water can help your body replace the salts it loses and keep you from getting

dehydrated, especially when you're losing a lot of fluids.

3. Stay away from sugary and fizzy drinks. People with ostomies may experience more gas and bloating when they drink these types of drinks.

To stay refreshed without feeling sick, choose low-sugar, non-carbonated drinks like herbal teas, infused water, and fruit juices that have been diluted.

4. Sip Throughout the Day: Instead of drinking a lot of fluids all at once, sip them slowly throughout the day to keep your digestive system from getting too full and to lower your risk of problems linked to your ostomy, like high output or leakage.

5. Watch Your pee Output: The color and amount of your pee can tell you how well you're drinking water. Pale yellow urine means you're drinking enough water, while dark yellow or amber pee could mean you're dehydrated and need to drink more water.

By using these hydration tips, people with ostomies can keep their fluid levels in check, help their bodies heal, and improve their general health.

Making smoothies is a great way for people with ostomies to stay refreshed and get important vitamins and nutrients. Whether you eat them as a meal replacement or as a healthy snack, energizing smoothies are a quick and tasty way to stay hydrated and get nutrients. Here are some drink recipes that are good for people with ostomies and will give them energy:

1. A smoothie called "Green Goddess" is very healthy because it has lots of veggies, leafy greens, and protein-rich ingredients. To make a treat that is both cool and energizing, blend spinach, kale, banana, Greek yogurt, almond milk, and a scoop of protein powder.

2. Berry Blast Smoothie: This berry blast smoothie is full of antioxidants and vitamins, which are great for the immune system and for helping the body heal after surgery. Berries like strawberries, blueberries, raspberries, spinach, avocado, almond milk, and a tablespoon of flaxseeds can all be mixed to make a tasty and healthy drink.

3. Tropical Paradise drink: This cool drink with pineapple, mango, coconut water, and a splash of lime juice will take you to a tropical paradise.

This tropical treat is full of vitamin C and fluids, so it will keep you hydrated and help you feel better.

4. Smoothie with Protein: This smoothie with protein is great for people who need an extra protein boost. You can make a healthy drink that will keep you full and fueled by blending banana, peanut butter, chocolate protein powder, spinach, and almond milk.

Ostomy patients can enjoy tasty and healthy drinks that help them heal and stay healthy for a long time by adding these energising smoothie recipes to their diet.

Patients with ostomies can stay refreshed and fed with a lot of different kinds of refreshing drinks besides smoothies. From herbal teas to flavored water, these drink ideas offer variety and keep you hydrated without sacrificing taste or health.

Here are some cool drink ideas for people with ostomies:

1. Herbal Teas: Peppermint, chamomile, and ginger are some examples of herbal teas that can quell stomach upset and keep you hydrated without adding sugar or caffeine. Warm herbal tea is a soothing and energising drink that you can enjoy after meals or during the day.

2. Infused Water: To add flavor and nutrients to plain water without adding extra calories or chemicals, infuse it with fresh fruits, veggies, and herbs. If you want a new way to stay hydrated, try

mixing cucumber and mint, lemon and ginger, or watermelon and basil.

3.Coconut Water: Since coconut water is naturally high in electrolytes, it is a great choice for ostomy patients who want to replace fluids they've lost and stay hydrated. You can drink coconut water by itself or add a tropical touch to smoothies and mocktails by making them with it.

4. Vegetable drinks: Vegetable drinks that are freshly squeezed are a great way to get a lot of vitamins, minerals, and antioxidants without all the fiber. Vegetables that are high in nutrients, like kale, spinach, carrots, and beets, can be added to juices to make them healthy and refreshing.

Ostomy patients can find new ways to stay hydrated and fed while enjoying a wide range of flavors and health benefits by trying these cool drink ideas.

drinks and smoothies are an important part of an ostomy patient's diet because they keep them hydrated, give them calories, and make them feel good. People with ostomies can stay properly hydrated, help their bodies heal, and improve their long-term health by following hydration tips, trying out energising smoothie recipes and looking for other cool drink ideas. Professionals in health care or registered dietitians can give you personalized dietary advice and suggestions based on your needs and tastes.

CHAPTER 8
MAKING PLANS FOR MEALS AND COOKING IN BULK

Planning meals and making them in large batches are important parts of eating well, especially for people who have an ostomy bag. These tips help make sure that you have a healthy, easy-to-follow diet that supports your general health and the ostomy works well. Planning and preparing meals ahead of time not only makes mealtimes easier but also helps digestion and nutrient intake, which is very important for people who are still getting used to life after surgery.

Tips for Planning Meals Efficiently:

Planning meals ahead of time is very important for sticking to an ostomy bag care diet. It means giving careful thought to dietary needs, personal tastes, and lifestyle factors.

To begin, it's important to talk to a doctor or a trained dietitian about making a meal plan that fits your specific needs.

This plan should focus on a range of nutrient-dense foods, like fruits, veggies, whole grains, healthy fats, lean proteins, and any food allergies or restrictions.

Making a weekly or monthly meal plan with breakfast, lunch, dinner, and snacks is a good way to stick to a diet. This calendar helps you keep track of your food lists and makes sure you get enough of all the nutrients your body needs. Including a variety of colors, tastes, and textures in your meals not only makes your senses happier, but also gives your body the vitamins, minerals, and enzymes it needs to heal and stay healthy.

Batch cooking is another way to plan meals efficiently. Making a lot of meals ahead of time can save people time and effort on busy days while still giving them access to healthy, ostomy-friendly choices.

Batch cooking lets you make a lot of soups, stews, casseroles, and other meals at once, which can then be easily divided up and saved for later use. Additionally, using versatile ingredients like quinoa, lentils, and beans lets you make a variety of meals that you can eat all week.

Tips for Cooking in Large Groups on Busy Days:
Batch cooking is especially helpful for people with busy lives because it cuts down on the need to make meals often and makes sure that healthy meals are always available. Set aside a day of the week, like Sunday, when you have more time to prepare meals, to do all of your cooking at once.

This will help you get the most done. This lets people focus on making and saving meals for the next week, which speeds up the process and makes daily life less stressful.

When making a lot of food at once, it's best to pick recipes that can be frozen and then reheated.

This keeps the quality of the meals over time and extends their shelf life. Soups, stews, chili, and pasta sauces are great for cooking in large amounts because they are easy to divide into serving sizes and store in containers or freezer bags that keep air out. Also, buying good storage cases that can go in the freezer and the microwave will make reheating meals more convenient and easier.

Adding different tastes and cuisines to batch-cooked meals keeps things interesting and encourages people to stick to a healthy diet. Adding different herbs, spices, and flavours to food gives it more depth and complexity, which makes it more enjoyable and filling. Using seasonal foods in meals not only makes them healthier, but it also helps local farmers and has less of an effect on the earth.

How to Freeze and Store Ostomy-Friendly Foods:

It is very important to freeze and store ostomy-friendly meals the right way to keep their quality and safety. It's important to let ready-made meals cool down before putting them in the freezer.

This stops ice crystals from forming and keeps the nutrients and taste of the food. To make sure there is proper movement and no waste, it's also a good idea to write on each container the date it was prepared and what's inside.

When keeping frozen meals, it's important to use containers or bags that can go in the freezer and seal tightly to keep food from freezing and getting contaminated. Soups, stews, and casseroles should be stored in glass containers with lids that fit tightly. Individual servings of pasta, grains, and veggies should be stored in freezer bags. It's best to leave some room at the top of bags or containers so that they can expand when they freeze. This will lower the chance of leaks or spills.

For the best safety and quality, frozen meals should be eaten within three to six months of being made, based on the type of food and how it was stored.

To stop bacteria from growing and foodborne diseases, it is important to safely thaw frozen meals. Meals should be thawed in the fridge overnight or defrosted in the microwave on the right setting for best results. To make sure food is safe, meals that have been frozen should be brought up to the right temperature before being eaten, which is usually 165°F (74°C).

To sum up, planning meals and cooking large amounts at once are very helpful for eating well and following an ostomy bag care diet correctly. People can make food preparation easier, save time and effort, and make sure they always have access to healthy, satisfying meals by using effective strategies and techniques. People can eat a varied and balanced diet that helps them heal, feel good, and stay healthy in the long run if they plan, prepare, and store their food properly.

CHAPTER 9
GOING OUT TO EAT AND TRAVELLING

Keeping a good diet and taking care of an ostomy bag at the same time can be hard, especially when going out to eat or travelling. But if you plan and are aware of what's going on, you can handle these situations with confidence and ease. The goal of this detailed guide is to give people with ostomies useful information and useful tips on how to stay healthy and eat well while traveling and eating out.

Feeling Good About Going Out to Eat

Going to a restaurant can be fun, but it can also be scary for people with ostomies because they don't know what to order and could be uncomfortable.

You can feel confident when you eat out, though, if you plan and know what to expect.

First, it's important to do research on restaurants ahead of time and pick ones that are known for being able to accommodate dietary restrictions or provide ostomy-friendly choices. When you order, choose foods that are well-cooked and easy to digest, like grilled proteins, steamed veggies, and plain grains, to lower your risk of digestive problems.

Also, talk to the server in private about any dietary needs or worries you have about your ostomy to make sure you have a smooth and comfortable meal.

Also, it's best to stay away from foods that are too spicy or greasy, as these can make stomach problems worse. Overall, going out to eat with an ostomy takes being proactive and communicating clearly to make sure a good experience.

Bringing Ostomy-Friendly Snacks on Trips

When you travel with an ostomy, you need to plan, especially for snacks and meals you can eat on the go. Bringing snacks that are safe for people with ostomies is important for keeping up your energy and avoiding feeling uncomfortable while traveling. Choose snacks that are easy to carry and don't go bad quickly, like whole-grain crackers, nuts, seeds, dried fruits, and raisins.

These snacks give you a mix of nutrients and fiber without making your stomach upset. Also, to lower the risk of problems related to your ostomy while you're traveling, you might want to bring individual servings of low-residue foods like rice cakes, plain popcorn, or granola bars.

Also, it's important to stay hydrated. Carry a water bottle that you can refill and stay away from sugary drinks and too much coffee, which can make you dehydrated and irritate your bowels.

People can travel easily and comfortably without worrying about their nutrition needs if they carefully choose and pack snacks that are safe for people with ostomies.

How to Stay Healthy While Travelling

For people with ostomies in particular, eating healthy while on the go requires careful planning and thoughtful food choices.

If you want to make sure you get enough nutrition and digestive comfort while traveling, try using these tips.

First, eat mostly whole, unprocessed foods like veggies, fruits, lean proteins, and whole grains. These foods give you all the nutrients you need and are good for your digestive health.

To keep from getting hungry or uncomfortable while traveling, bring a variety of snacks and meals that are easy on the stomach, like yogurt, smoothies, boiled eggs, and cooked veggies.

Also, watch your portions and don't eat too much; this can put stress on your gut system and cause gas or bloating.

When you eat out at restaurants or fast food chains, pick foods that are low in fat, sugar, and salt, and try to get them grilled or steamed whenever you can. Lastly, pay attention to your body's signals and make changes as needed to make sure you can eat comfortably and enjoyably while you're on the go.

People with ostomies can eat a healthy, balanced diet even when they are traveling or eating out if they follow these tips.

CHAPTER 10
HOW TO DEAL WITH PROBLEMS

Having ostomy surgery can make a big difference in a person's life, both physically and mentally. Getting through these problems takes a multifaceted approach that includes things like dealing with food intolerances and digestive pain and looking for help and resources. By taking care of all of these things, people can better adjust to their new lifestyle after surgery, which is good for their health and well-being.

How to Deal with Digestive Pain:

Taking care of digestive pain is one of the main worries for people who have an ostomy bag. After surgery, the digestive system goes through a lot of changes that can cause problems like gas, bloating, and irregular bowel movements. To ease these symptoms, it is important to make changes to your food that are specific to your needs.

This could mean eating smaller meals more often to make digestion easier and keep the GI system from having to work too hard. Also, eating fiber-rich foods like fruits, veggies, and whole grains can help you stay regular and avoid constipation, which is a common problem for people with ostomies.

Also, staying hydrated is important for keeping your gut system working well. Drinking enough water keeps you from getting dehydrated and helps stools move easily through the digestive system. But people should be careful about what drinks they drink. They should choose water and electrolyte-rich drinks over-caffeinated and carbonated drinks, which can make stomach problems worse.

Also, it's important to keep an eye on your food and make changes based on your tolerance levels.

Some people may have stomach problems when they eat certain foods, so they need to avoid them or eat them in moderation.

Keeping a food log can help you figure out what might be causing your symptoms and make changes to your diet to address them. Additionally, talking to a qualified dietitian who specializes in ostomy care can give you personalised advice and help you healthily deal with digestive discomfort.

How to Deal with Food Intolerances:

People who have an ostomy bag also have to deal with food intolerances, which can be hard. A lot of people may become more sensitive to certain foods after surgery, which can cause stomach problems like bloating, cramps, and diarrhea. To reduce pain and improve gut health, it's important to know what foods cause problems and stay away from them.

To find specific food intolerances, an elimination diet may be suggested. This means cutting out common trigger foods like dairy, gluten, and high-fat foods for a while and then slowly adding them back in while watching for bad responses.

Adding fermented foods like yogurt and kefir to your diet can also help keep your gut healthy and may help some people with stomach problems.

Mindful eating can also help people who have trouble with food intolerances. To do this, you need to pay attention to signs of hunger and fullness, chew your food well, and eat in a calm setting. Avoiding big meals, especially right before bed, can also help your general health and make you less likely to have stomach pain.

Looking for Help and Resources:

People who have an ostomy bag may find it hard to get through life, but they don't have to do it alone. Support from healthcare professionals, support groups, and internet communities can be very helpful. They can offer advice, support, and friendship. Nurses, dietitians, and ostomy experts are some of the health professionals who can give you personalised advice on how to care for your ostomy, make changes to your diet, and deal with stress.

You can get mental support and useful tips for living with an ostomy by joining a support group or getting in touch with people who have been through similar things. You can share your stories, ask questions, and find a lot of information about ostomy care and management on online forums and social media sites.

Keeping people informed about resources like educational materials, workshops, and counseling services can also give them the power to play an active part in their recovery and long-term health. People who are proactive about getting help and resources can improve their quality of life, learn new ways to deal with problems, and do well even though living with an ostomy can be hard.

CHAPTER 11

QUESTIONS PEOPLE OFTEN ASK

People who have had ostomy surgery often have to make big changes to their lives, including what they eat. It is very important for people who have had surgery to understand the ins and outs of the ostomy bag care diet. This part answers some of the most common questions about the ostomy bag care diet by giving you expert advice and tips for the best management.

Questions People Ask About the Ostomy Bag Maintenance Diet

People who have had ostomy surgery often have questions about what they can eat and how they can best take care of their ostomy bags while still eating well and staying healthy overall. One of the biggest worries is figuring out which foods are safe to eat and which ones could cause problems like clogs or too much gas production.

People may also ask about ways to keep the area around the stoma from smelling, leaking, and getting irritated. There may also be questions about how food affects the consistency and frequency of stoma output, as well as how to change eating habits to cause the least amount of pain or trouble.

Figuring these things out requires a complex approach that includes not only learning about how different foods affect the digestive system physiologically but also learning how to care for and maintain an ostomy. To give people the information and confidence to properly take care of their ostomy, it's important to address all of their concerns.

Tips and advice from experts

Talking to medical professionals, especially registered dietitians who specialize in ostomy care, can give you very useful advice that is tailored to your specific needs and tastes. These experts can give you personalized food advice based on things like the type of ostomy surgery you had (ileostomy, colostomy, or urostomy), your health conditions, the medicines you take, and your lifestyle.

A well-balanced, varied, and easily digestible eating plan is one of the most important parts of an ostomy bag care diet. Fruits, vegetables, lean proteins, whole grains, and healthy fats are some examples of whole foods that have been minimally processed and are high in important nutrients.

But it's important to make changes to your diet slowly so that your digestive system has time to get used to the new foods and you can figure out which foods might make you sick.

Fiber intake is another important thing to think about because it can change the structure and length of your stools. People who have had colostomies can keep their bowel movements regular and avoid constipation by eating enough fiber-rich foods like fruits, veggies, whole grains, and legumes.

On the other hand, people who have ileostomies may need to limit the amount of fiber they eat to avoid having too much stool and possible clogs.

Staying hydrated is important for both keeping your ostomy working well and staying healthy in general. Making sure you drink enough water helps keep you from becoming dehydrated, which can make stools thicker and raise the risk of clogs. Promoting proper hydration can be done by telling people to drink water throughout the day and drinking less dehydrating drinks like coffee and wine.

Along with what you eat, making sure you take care of your ostomy bag properly is important for keeping it comfortable and giving you confidence. This includes removing and replacing the ostomy pouch regularly and making sure there is a tight seal around the stoma to stop leaks. Using ostomy devices like barrier rings or stoma paste can help the skin around the ostomy stay in place and avoid getting irritated.

Also, people should be aware of any possible allergens or irritants in ostomy goods or skin care products that are put on the peristomal area. Choosing hypoallergenic goods that don't have any scents and doing patch tests before using them can help lower the risk of bad reactions.

Teaching people about typical problems that come with ostomy surgery, like controlling gas and smells, can also give them the power to take action to solve these problems. Avoiding foods that cause gas, using ostomy deodorizers or pouch filters, and being careful about how you throw away your pouches can help ease these worries and improve your quality of life.

In the end, getting the best diet and ostomy care after surgery requires a mix of knowledge, practical skills, and ongoing support from medical experts and peer support groups.

People who have an ostomy can confidently and successfully go through life by getting answers to common questions, getting expert help, and working together to manage their ostomy.

CONCLUSION

Getting through the days after surgery with an ostomy bag takes both strength and careful planning of what you eat. You now have the tools, information, and recipes you need to make the most of your post-surgery diet for long-term health thanks to the complete guide.

Each part was carefully written to help you on your way to healing, from learning the basics of ostomy care to making meals that are safe for people with ostomies that are also good for you. This guide has many different recipes and food ideas that you can use to make the right choices for your needs, whether you want to start the day with a healthy breakfast, eat a filling lunch or dinner, or treat yourself to some guilt-free snacks and desserts.

No longer do big events and social gatherings have to be scary. Now you can find party recipes and planning tips that let you enjoy every moment without having to worry about your food needs.

You can also stick to your diet goals even if you are traveling or have a busy lifestyle by learning how to plan your meals, cook in bulk, and eat out with confidence.

Although you're on this journey, it's important to be aware of and deal with any problems that may come up, like stomach pain, food allergies, or finding help and resources. This guide's expert advice and tips will help you get past these problems and keep your general health in good shape.

Always keep in mind that you are not alone as you continue to heal. You have everything you need to live a full life with an ostomy bag: information, tasty recipes, and a group of people who care about you.